Stomal Therapy

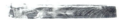

ROBYN SHELL at the time of writing this book was
senior stomal therapy nurse at the Repatriation
General Hospital, Concord. She is a past president
(1982) of the New South Wales branch of the
Australian Association of Stomal Therapy Nurses and
a member of the World Council of Enterostomal
Therapists.

DR E. LESLIE BOKEY is a senior lecturer in surgery at
the University of Sydney and a member of the Colon
and Rectal Department of the Repatriation General
Hospital, Concord.

Stomal Therapy

A Guide for Nurses, Practitioners and Patients

E.L. Bokey & Robyn Shell

PERGAMON PRESS

Sydney • Oxford • New York • Toronto • Paris • Frankfurt

This book is dedicated to Tami, Adam and Christopher

Pergamon Press (Australia) Pty Ltd,
19a Boundary Street, Rushcutters Bay, N.S.W. 2011, Australia.

Pergamon Press Ltd,
Headington Hill Hall, Oxford OX3 0BW, England.

Pergamon Press Inc.,
Maxwell House, Fairview Park, Elmsford, N.Y. 10523, U.S.A.

Pergamon Press Canada Ltd,
Suite 104, 150 Consumers Road, Willowdale, Ontario M2J 1P9, Canada.

Pergamon Press GmbH,
6242 Kronberg-Taunus, Hammerweg 6, Postfach 1305, Federal Republic of Germany.

Pergamon Press SARL,
24 rue des Ecoles, 75240 Paris, Cedex 05, France.

First published 1985

Copyright © 1985 E.L. Bokey & Robyn Shell

Cover design by Robert Taylor
Typeset in Australia by Comset Pty Ltd, Melbourne
Printed in Singapore by Singapore National Printers

National Library of Australia Cataloguing in Publication Data:

Bokey, E.L. (Eli Leslie), 1946-.
    Stomal therapy.

    ISBN 0 08 029862 1 (flexi).
    ISBN 0 08 029865 6 (hard).

    1. Enterostomy. 2. Postoperative care. 3. Ostomates
    Rehabilitation. I. Shell, Robyn. II. Title.

617'.554

Contents

Foreword   vii

Acknowledgements   ix

List of Terms   xi

Introduction   xiii

1. Indications for a Stoma   1

2. Siting a Stoma   24

3. Immediate Post-Operative Care of a Stoma   30

4. Management of an End Sigmoid Colostomy   40

5. Management of an Ileostomy   59

6. The Continent Ileostomy   73

7. Temporary Stomata   81

8. Urinary Diversion Stomas   89

9. Quality of Life   101

Foreword

The provision of an artificial stoma is necessary in the treatment of a variety of diseases; either temporarily as part of a staged surgical procedure, or permanently when the natural outlet and sphincter mechanism cannot be preserved. In either case it is a devastating concept for the patient.

The technique of fashioning stomas and their subsequent management has undergone dramatic improvement during the last thirty years. Prior to this, stomas were regarded with abhorrence by surgeons, nursing staff and patients alike.

This book is timely. It is written in simple language with simple illustrations which help surgeons, general practitioners, and nursing staff to bring up to date their management of stomas. Many of these practitioners both nursing and medical will have received their training prior to the development of new techniques and the advent of the stoma therapy nurse. This book will provide an easy reference to enable them to help their patients' particular problems.

M.T. PHEILS
Emeritus Professor of Surgery
University of Sydney

Acknowledgements

We wish to thank the Colostomy Rehabilitation Association of N.S.W., the Ileostomy Association of N.S.W. and E. R. Squibb and Sons Pty Ltd for their help and support with this project. We would also like to thank Emeritus Professor M. T. Pheils, Mr M. K. Killingback, Mr P. H. Chapuis, Sister H. Hill and Mr P. O. W. Maher for their constructive help and criticism. Mr J. Meyer was responsible for many of the illustrations and Mr R. Hansen (Department of Illustration, Repatriation General Hospital) provided his able services. Finally, we would like to thank the medical and nursing administration of the Repatriation General Hospital Concord, for their help and support.

List of Terms

ANASTOMOSIS is the joining by sutures or staples of two intestinal segments.

ANASTOMOTIC LEAK is a defect in an anastomosis which allows the escape of bowel contents into the peritoneal cavity.

RESECTION is the excision of some portion of the intestine.

ANTERIOR RESECTION refers to excision of the rectum (but not the anus) and anastomosis of the colon to the rectal stump.

PROXIMAL AND DISTAL refers to the position of a segment of bowel relative to the mouth. Distal is further away from the mouth and proximal is closer to the mouth. Thus, the anus is distal to the rectum, which is distal to the sigmoid colon. In turn, the ileum is proximal to the caecum which is proximal to the transverse colon.

Introduction

A stoma usually refers to the exteriorisation of a segment of the gastro-intestinal or urinary tract onto the abdomen. The excreta then has to be collected from the stoma into an appliance and disposed of.

This procedure is viewed by most people as being very unpleasant and distasteful. It is therefore not surprising that many patients look upon the prospect of living for the rest of their lives with a permanent abdominal wall stoma with fear and anxiety. A poor understanding of our own anatomy and physiology, and our reluctance to discuss in detail bodily functions such as defaecation, unfortunately only adds to this fear.

Continence (or control over our excreta) for most of us is taken for granted and the thought of losing this control causes anxiety and distress to most patients who are faced with the prospect of a stoma. These fears are accentuated by the stress of ill health which often accompanies the disease for which the stoma is necessary. These patients therefore not only have to accept a change in their body image and function, but they also have to contend with chronic illness and the stress of major abdominal surgery.

In the past, stomas earned a bad reputation because of inadequate surgical techniques, lack of suitable appliances, and the absence of stomal care and self-help groups. All these factors combined to make life with a stoma difficult and impractical. Ostomates would often not leave their houses for fear of accidental leakage and social embarrassment. They would often become reclusive and would consider themselves unsuitable for work, marriage or social intercourse. Because of the lack of an integrated team approach, patients would frequently get their information in fragments which further added to their confusion.

Over the past thirty years, however, dramatic improvements have occured and these have revolutionised the ostomate's lifestyle. Although advances in surgical techniques have contributed, the most significant contributions, however, have been made by the development of modern disposable appliances, and by the emergence of stomal therapy as a specialised nursing discipline. Furthermore, self-help organisations have been formed in every major city and these have offered the prospective ostomate information and a forum for discussion.

Today most ostomates enjoy a fully active social and working life, and the majority feel that their initial anxieties were in the end not justified.

CHAPTER 1

Indications for a Stoma

INTRODUCTION

Stoma is Greek for mouth. When a segment of intestine is exteriorised to the abdominal wall, it is referred to as a stoma. There are several million people in the world who have a stoma, and they are frequently referred to as ostomates.

The name given to a particular stoma depends on which segment of intestine is exteriorised. For example, a gastrostomy refers to exteriorisation of the stomach; jejunostomy of the jejunum, that is the upper end of the small intestine (Figure 1.1); ileostomy of the ileum, that is the lower end of the small intestine (Figure 1.2); colostomy of the colon (Figure 1.3); and caecostomy of the caecum.

The large intestine, or colon, includes the caecum, the ascending and transverse colon, the descending and sigmoid colon, the rectum and the anal canal (Figure 1.4). The term 'procto' refers to the rectum and the anal canal.

Small intestinal fluid is non-odourous, and contains activated enzymes which may excoriate the skin. It is more copious from a jejunostomy than an ileostomy. Approximately 500 ml per day are excreted from an established ileostomy. The consistency of faeces from a colostomy depends on which segment of colon is exteriorised. It is fluid from a caecostomy but it becomes thicker the closer the stoma is to the anus.

1

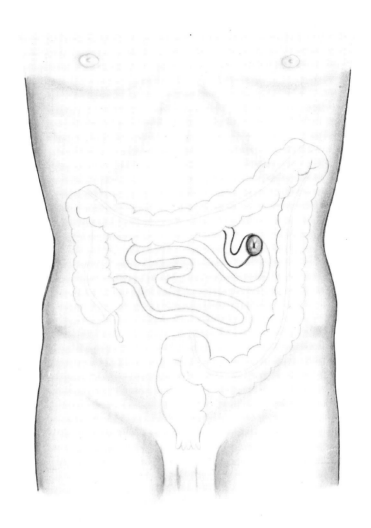

Fig. 1.1   Jejunostomy

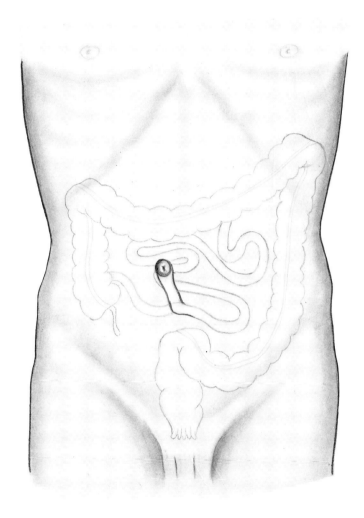

Fig. 1.2   Ileostomy

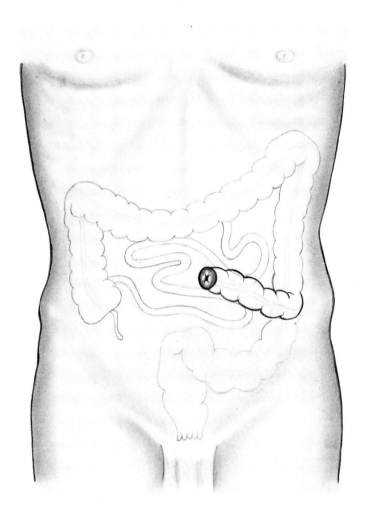

Fig. 1.3   Colostomy

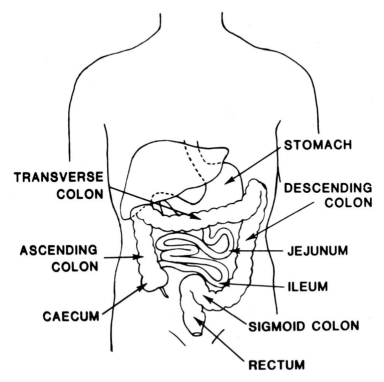

Fig. 1.4   Anatomy of the intestine

CONDITIONS FOR WHICH A STOMA MAY BE NECESSARY

Carcinoma of the colon and rectum
This is the commonest internal malignancy in both sexes in Western society.

Ulcerative colitis
This is an inflammatory condition of the large intestine which affects all of the colon from the anus to the caecum. It involves the mucosal layer of the bowel and occurs predominantly in young females. It may predispose to colonic carcinoma.

Crohn's disease

This is an inflammatory condition which may affect any portion of the gastrointestinal tract, from the mouth to the anus. It involves the whole thickness of the bowel wall and occurs predominately in young adults.

Diverticular disease of the colon

In this condition, which affects the sigmoid colon in particular, the mucosa herniates through the muscular layer of the bowel wall. These pockets or 'diverticulae' may become inflamed causing diverticulitis.

Injury to the intestine

In some instances of injury, especially when the colon is involved, exteriorisation of the affected segments may be necessary.

Familial polyposis coli

This is a hereditary abnormality in which there are multiple polyps in the colon and rectum. There is an associated high incidence of malignancy.

Volvulus

In this condition a segment of bowel, usually the sigmoid colon, rotates on itself, endangering its blood supply and causing obstruction.

COMMON SURGICAL PROCEDURES INVOLVING A STOMA

Elective surgery (non-urgent)

1. *Abdominal-perineal excision (A.P.E.) of the rectum and the anal canal, and end colostomy*
   PRINCIPLE INDICATIONS: Carcinoma of the lower rectum and anal canal.

   The rectum, anal canal and anus are resected (Figure 1.5) and an end colostomy fashioned (Figure 1.6).

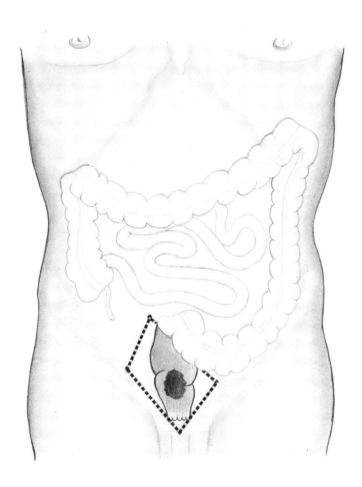

Fig. 1.5 A.P.E. of rectum and anus

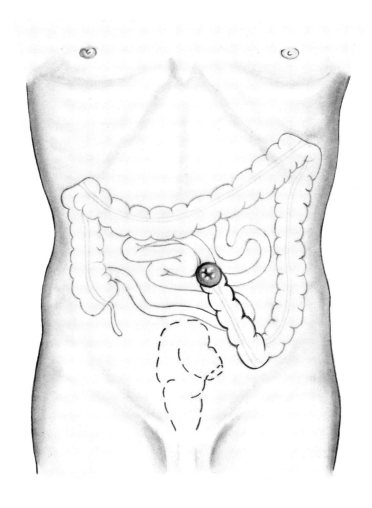

Fig. 1.6   A.P.E.: end-colostomy fashioned

2. *Total proctocolectomy and end ileostomy*
   PRINCIPLE INDICATIONS: Ulcerative colitis, familial polyposis coli and Crohn's disease.

   The entire colon, rectum and anus are resected (Figure 1.7) and an end ileostomy fashioned (Figure 1.8).

3. *Left-sided colonic resection (including anterior resection) and defuctioning loop transverse colostomy*
   PRINCIPLE INDICATIONS: A left-sided colonic lesion such as carcinoma or diverticular disease.

   A colostomy is used in this instance to minimise the consequences of a possible anastomotic leak. Faeces from this proximal lumen of the colostomy is diverted into an appliance, away from the anastomosis. The lesion is resected (Figure 1.9). The free ends are anastomosed and a loop transverse colostomy supported by a rod is exteriorised. The main incision is closed and the loop opened to establish a colostomy (Figure 1.10). The colostomy is usually closed several weeks later when the anastomosis has healed satisfactorily (Figure 1.11).

Emergency surgery

1. *Laparotomy and loop transverse colostomy*
   PRINCIPLE INDICATIONS: Distal obstruction (secondary to carcinoma or diverticular disease), distal perforation or injury.

   The transverse colostomy in this instance diverts faeces away from the site of obstruction or injury. A laparotomy is performed and the diagnosis confirmed. To make a transverse colostomy a loop of transverse colon supported by a rod is exteriorised (Figure 1.12) and opened in the operating room (Figure 1.13), after the main incision has been closed

   At a later date, the diseased segment is resected and a third operation is required to close the transverse colostomy. This is known as a three-stage procedure.

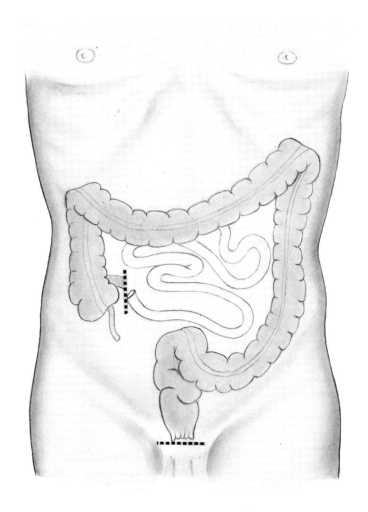

Fig. 1.7   Procto-colectomy

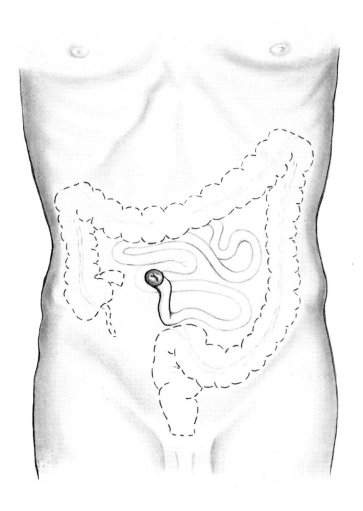

Fig. 1.8   Procto-colectomy: End-ileostomy following
resection of colon, rectum and anus

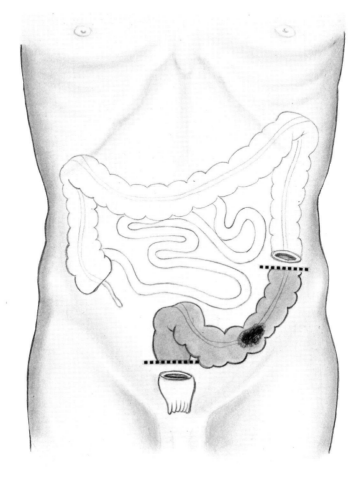

Fig. 1.9 Carcinoma of sigmoid colon resected

Fig. 1.10 (a) Free ends anastomosed and loop of transverse colon exteriorised and supported by rod

(b) Detail of exteriorised transverse colon supported by rod

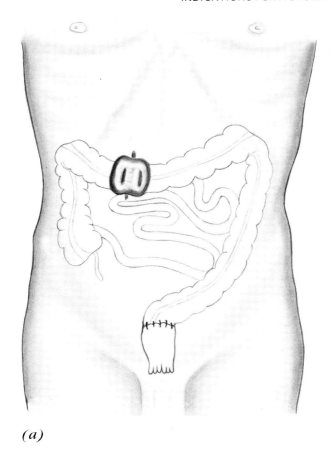

(a)

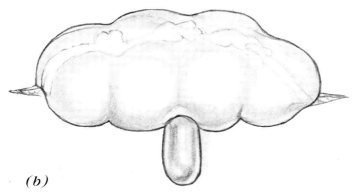

(b)

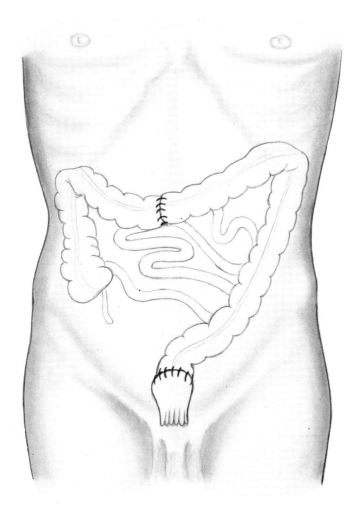

Fig. 1.11   Colostomy closed

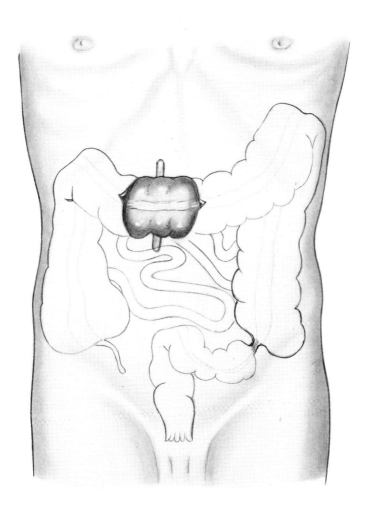

Fig. 1.12   Obstructed lesion: loop transverse colostomy

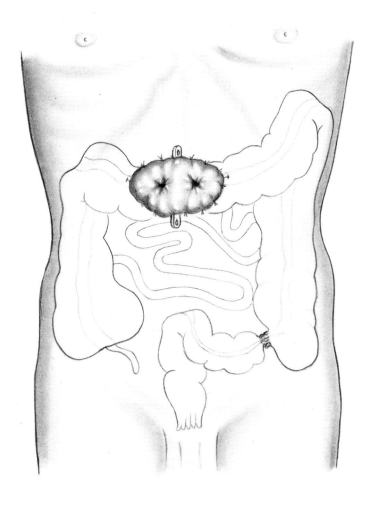

Fig. 1.13   Colostomy opened after closing main wound

2. *Laparotomy and caecostomy*
   PRINCIPLE INDICATIONS: Distal obstruction, secondary to carcinoma or diverticular disease. In some patients in whom there is distal obstruction, the surgeon may elect to do a caecostomy to divert the faeces (Figure 1.14).

3. *Resection without anastomosis*
   PRINCIPLE INDICATIONS: Sigmoid volvulus, perforated sigmoid diverticulitis, colonic injury.

   In some instances if there is undue risk in performing an immediate resection and anastomosis, the surgeon may elect to resect the diseased segment (Figure 1.15) and exteriorise both the proximal and distal ends. In this instance the proximal stoma is functioning, and the defunctioned stoma which secretes mucous is known as a mucous fistula (Figure 1.16).
   Alternatively, the distal end may be oversewn and left in the pelvis in which case the procedure is referred to as a Hartmann's procedure (Figure 1.17).

TECHNIQUE OF MAKING A STOMA

At the selected site, a disc of skin and subcutaneous tissue is excised (Figure 1.18). The dissection is deepended through the rectus muscle into the peritoneal cavity to comfortably fit two fingers (Figure 1.19). The segment of bowel is exteriorised and sutured to the skin. A colostomy should be just above skin level (Figure 1.20). However, with an ileostomy, the ileum is exteriorised for three inches and everted so that it may protrude into an appliance, thereby preventing contact between excoriating ileal fluid and the skin (Figure 1.21).

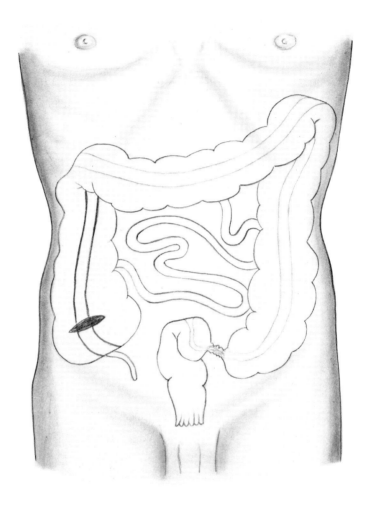

Fig. 1.14 Obstructive lesion: diversion by caecostomy

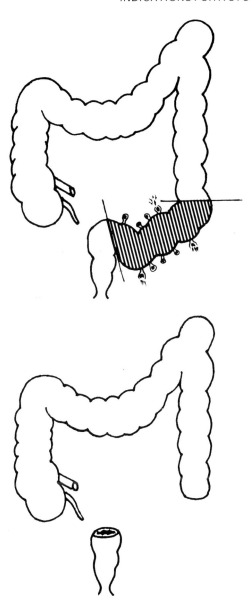

Fig. 1.15 Perforated diverticulitis. Segment resected without anastomosis

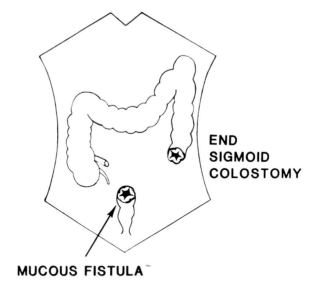

END
SIGMOID
COLOSTOMY

MUCOUS FISTULA

Fig. 1.16 Both ends exteriorised

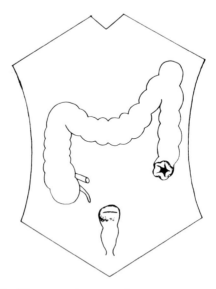

Fig. 1.17 Hartmann's procedure: rectum oversewn,
not exteriorised

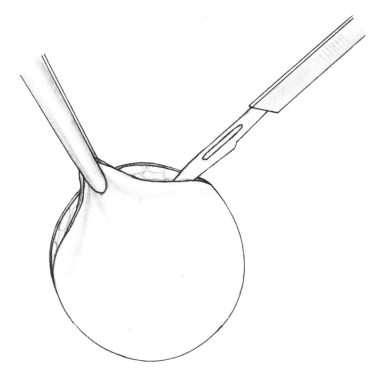

Fig. 1.18   Disc excised

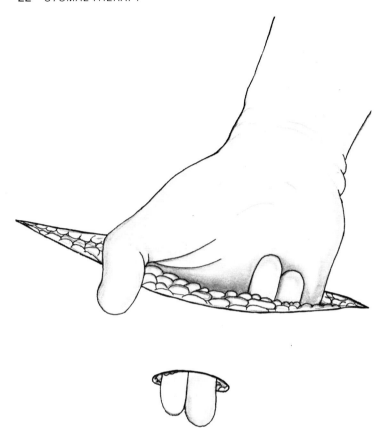

Fig. 1.19 Opening into abdominal wall opposite selected site

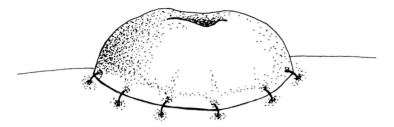

Fig. 1.20   Colostomy

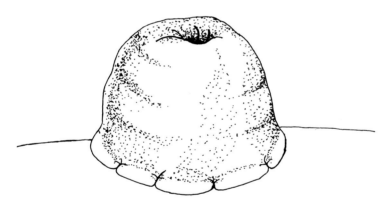

Fig. 1.21   Ileostomy

CHAPTER 2

Siting a Stoma

A stoma should be correctly sited pre-operatively to achieve optimum post-operative management. The stomal therapy nurse, the patient and the surgeon together choose the most appropriate site, which should be as close to the midline as the incision allows. It should also be opposite the rectus muscle and away from scars, bony prominences, skin folds, depressions, and if possible away from the belt line. Furthermore, it should be within sight and reach of the patient.

Siting should be performed while the patient lies, sits, bends and stands to ensure that all positions are taken into account. Attention should be directed not only to the patient's present build but to anticipated post-operative weight changes.

It is common to use a disc the diameter of which is similar to the adherent surface of the pouch and to indicate the site with a permanent marking pen.

SITING AN END SIGMOID COLOSTOMY

Three lines are drawn A-A midline, B-B lateral edge of the rectus muscle, C-C umbilical crease (Figure 2.1). The disc is placed so that its edges touch A-A and B-B (Figure 2.2).

The patient sits up, and corrections are made to ensure that the stoma is not situated between fat folds, and is easily accessible to the patient (Figure 2.3). The site is further checked with the patient standing and bending.

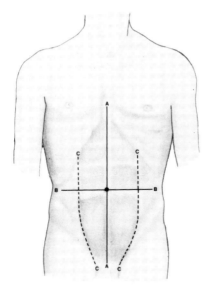

Fig. 2.1 Anatomical outlines for siting a stoma

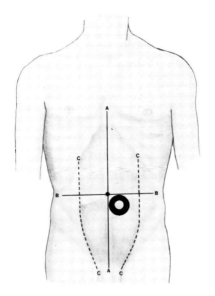

Fig. 2.2 Siting end sigmoid colostomy

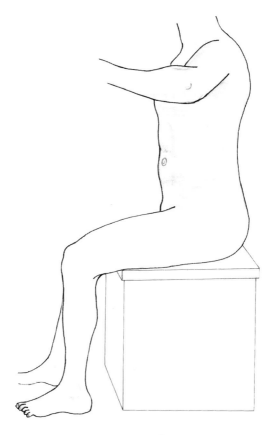

Fig. 2.3   Patient seated for accurate siting

SITING AN END ILEOSTOMY

Lines are drawn as shown in Figure 2.4 and the disc is applied to the right-lower quadrant.

SITING A TRANSVERSE COLOSTOMY

The disc is placed as shown in Figure 2.5. Particular care is taken to ensure that the disc does not encroach on the costal margin especially when the patient sits or bends.

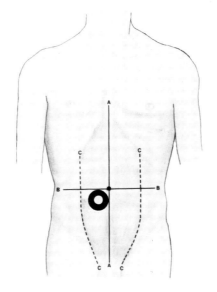

Fig. 2.4   Siting an end ileostomy

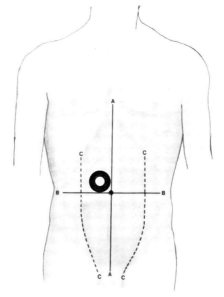

Fig. 2.5   Siting a transverse colostomy

SITING A STOMA IN AN OBESE PATIENT

It is important to sit and stand the obese patient when siting a stoma. Securing an appliance may be difficult if the stoma is sited between two fat folds (Figure 2.6) or when obscured by a fat apron (Figure 2.7), consequently, a stoma should be sited on the summit of a fat fold and certainly above the lower edge of a fat apron.

SITING A STOMA IN A VERY THIN PATIENT

These patients have a scaphoid shaped abdomen and special care has to be taken to site the stoma away from depressions and bony prominences (Figure 2.8).

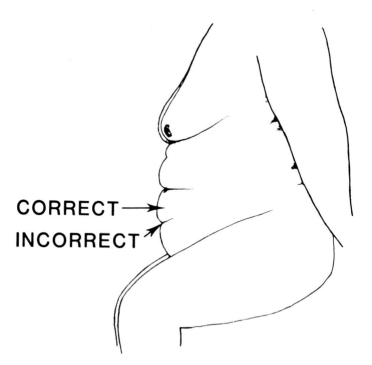

CORRECT→
INCORRECT

Fig. 2.6 Siting in an obese patient

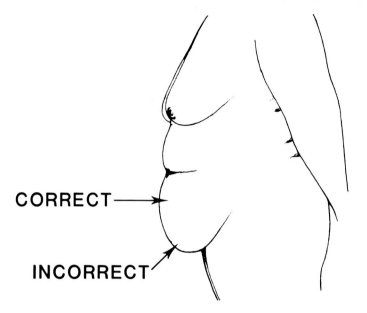

CORRECT———→

INCORRECT

Fig. 2.7   Siting in a patient with a fat apron

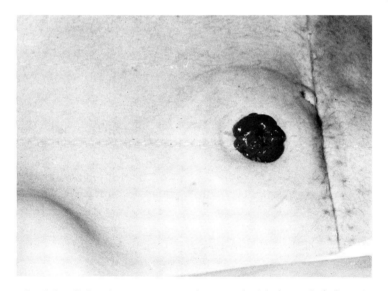

Fig. 2.8   Siting in a patient with a scaphoid shaped abdomen

CHAPTER 3

Immediate Post-Operative Care of a Stoma

OBSERVATION

All stomas should be observed regularly for colour and signs of retraction. The colour should be pink to dark red indicating viability (Colour Plate 1). Oedema may be present (Colour Plate 2) and usually resolves without specific treatment. A submucosal haematoma may occur and must not be confused with a necrotic stoma (Colour Plate 3). If any doubt exists about the viability of a stoma then the patient should be reviewed as soon as possible. Necrosis may be due to tension or inadequate blood supply, and usually necessitates urgent reoperation.

APPLICATION OF AN APPLIANCE POST-OPERATIVELY

After completing the procedure in the operating room the surgeon applies a pouch over the stoma. Several pouches may be suitable, however the folowing principles should be adhered to when making a selection. The appliance should have a backing which provides skin protection and is easy to remove without undue pain in the post-operative period. Karaya gum or Stomahesive backed pouches are therefore suitable. Furthermore, the pouch must be made of clear plastic to enable frequent observation of the stoma.

Within two to five days it will become necessary to change the appliance. Three different types are commonly used, and

30

the procedure varies according to the type of appliance chosen.

Skin protective wafer (e.g. Stomahesive) and adhesive pouch

The skin is washed with warm water only and dried. A pattern of the stoma is then made as shown in Figures 3.1 to 3.4. A skin protective wafer is cut to size using the pattern in Figure 3.5.

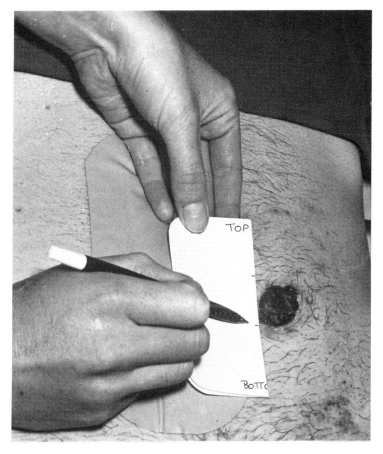

Figs. 3.1 to 3.4   Pattern of stoma being made

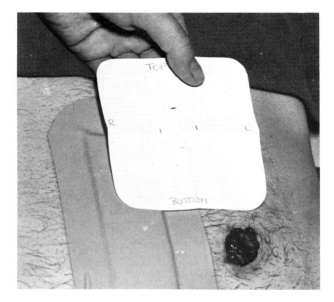

Fig. 3.2

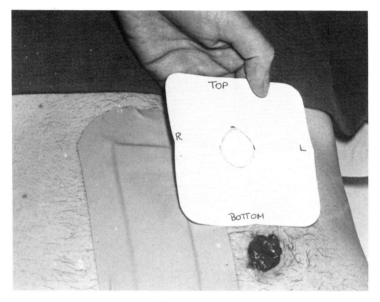

Fig. 3.3

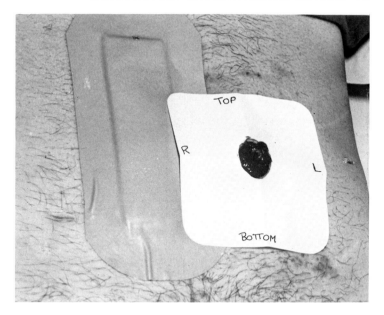

Fig. 3.4

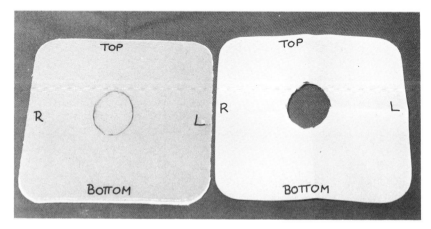

Fig. 3.5 Skin protective wafer: pattern outlined

A clear and drainable pouch with adhesive backing (Figure 3.6) is now prepared. An aperture with a diameter larger than that in the skin protective wafer is cut out. This is important so as to avoid leakage between the wafer and the adhesive on the pouch. The pouch is then pressed firmly against the wafer (Figure 3.7). The appliance may need to be trimmed away from the incision so as not to impinge on it. It is then pressed directly around the stoma to obtain a seal (Figure 3.8).

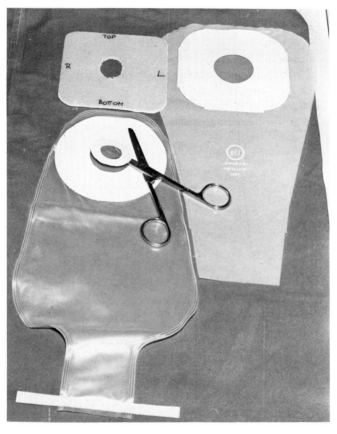

Fig. 3.6   Pouch with adhesive backing

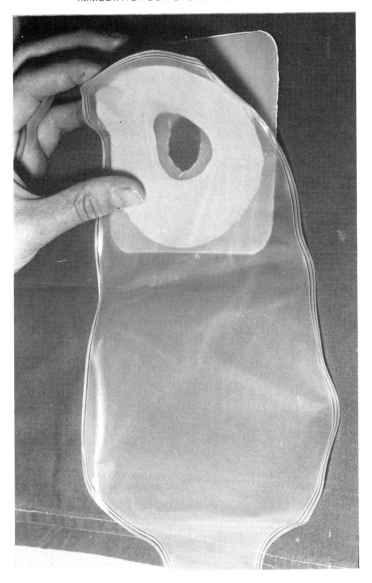

Fig. 3.7 Apply pouch to wafer

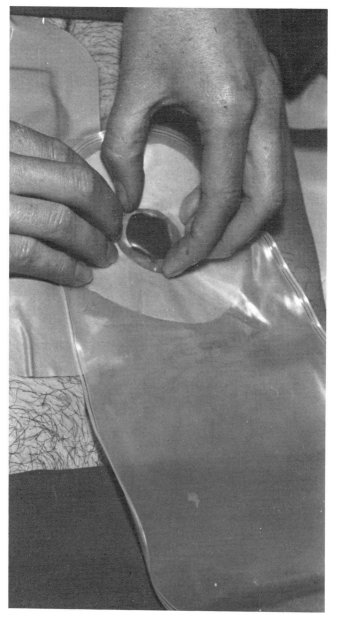

Fig. 3.8 Pouch and wafer applied over stoma

Karaya gum backed appliance

The aperture of the pouch is cut to size (Figure 3.9), the karaya gum is moistened slightly and the pouch is applied.

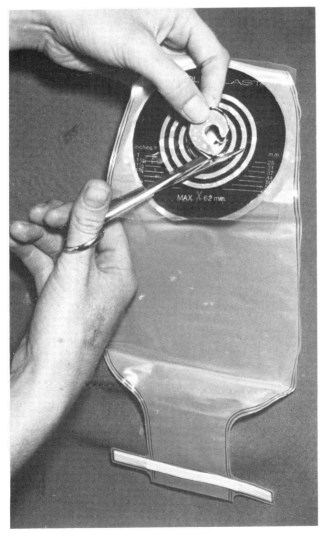

Fig. 3.9 Karaya gum appliance cut to size

Two piece appliances (e.g. Squibb System II)

A pattern of the stoma is made as described. A corresponding aperture is made in the base wafer which is then adhered to the skin (Figure 3.10). The pouch is then clipped into place (Figure 3.11).

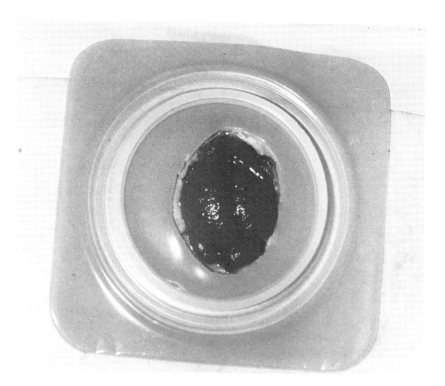

Fig. 3.10 Two-piece appliance: wafer base

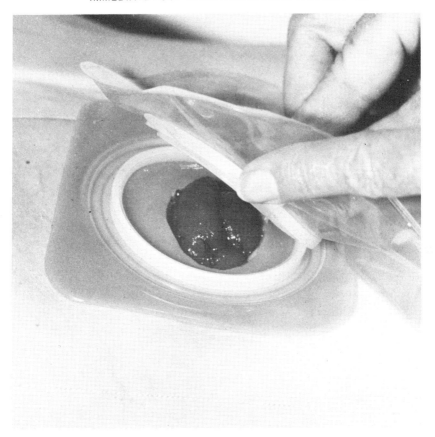

Fig. 3.11   Two-piece appliance: pouch clipped on

CHAPTER 4

Management of an End Sigmoid Colostomy

When the patient resumes a full diet, the faeces usually thickens and a change is made to a permanent appliance. The stomal therapy nurse and patient choose the most suitable pouch taking into account the patient's dexterity and mental acuity. Many appliances are available to suit individual build and preference. Although disposable appliances are favoured by many, some patients prefer to use semi-disposable ones.

Disposable Appliances

Many types of disposable appliances are available. Basically they vary according to the aperture, the colour, shape, texture and backing. It is difficult to list all the available appliances, however, some examples are given below to illustrate how particular types are used.

1. Pouches with a pre-cut aperture (Figure 4.1) may be desirable for patients with poor eyesight or arthritic fingers.
2. Pouches with a malleable backing (Figure 4.2) may be selected in obese patients with many skin folds so as to enable the pouch to conform to body contours.
3. A lightweight smaller pouch (Figure 4.3) may be preferred by an otherwise fit, active person.
4. Pouches incorporating a skin protective barrier (Figure 4.4) may be desirable for a person with delicate or excoriated skin.

Air vents and charcoal filters

These may be either incorporated in a disposable pouch, or small air vents may be made by the patient who may then elect to cover these with a disposable charcoal filter.

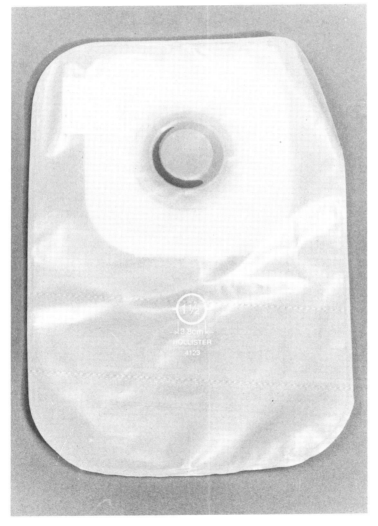

Fig. 4.1 Colostomy pouch: precut aperture

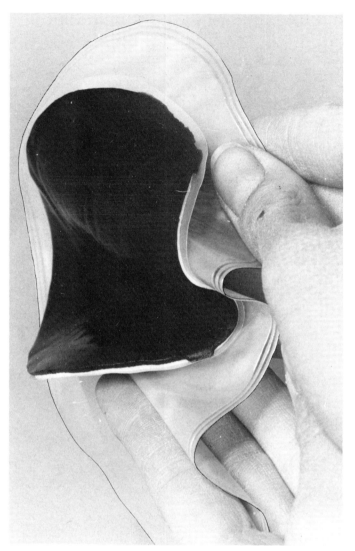

Fig. 4.2   Colostomy pouch: malleable backing

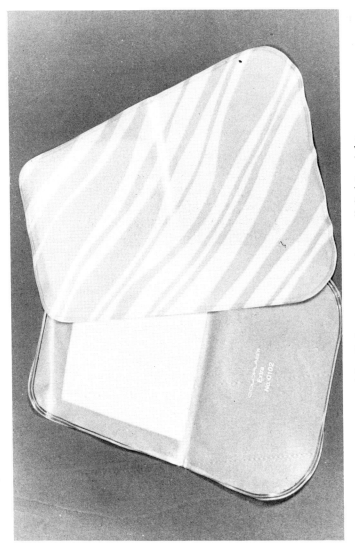

Fig. 4.3   Colostomy pouch: small, lightweight

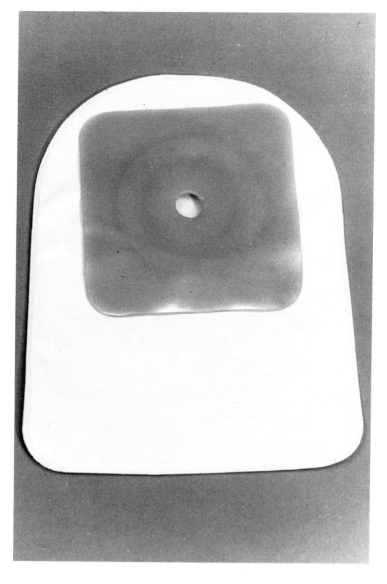

Fig. 4.4 Colostomy pouch incorporating protective barrier

SEMI-DISPOSABLE APPLIANCES

These usually consist of a flange (Figure 4.5) onto which a disposable plastic pouch is fitted. The flange is fixed to the peristomal skin using an adhesive with or without a skin barrier.

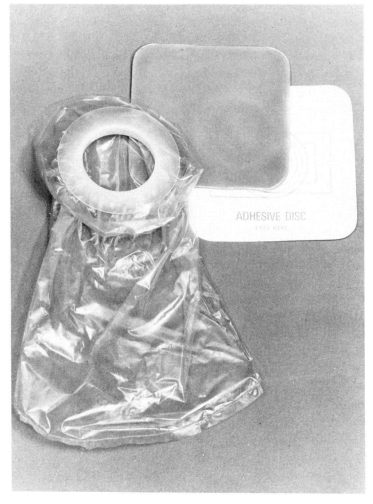

Fig. 4.5   Semidisposable appliance

GENERAL PRINCIPLES OF APPLYING A COLOSTOMY BAG

Stomal care should preferably be taught in a room which has a toilet and mirror, and which is separate from the general ward area.

All necessary equipment should be laid out systematically before commencing. The pouch aperture should be cut to size if a precut appliance is not used. The dirty pouch is gently peeled off using warm water or a weak solvent. After the colostomy is cleansed with tissue the patient may have a shower, and the new pouch is applied to the dried skin. The patient may either sit or stand and may find it helpful to use a mirror. It is important to stretch any skin creases before application to ensure a secure fit.

COLOSTOMY IRRIGATION

Irrigation is another method of managing a colostomy whereby a degree of continence may be achieved. The proximal colon is regularly irrigated with water thus enabling the patient to wear minimal protection between washouts. Irrigation is reserved for patients who have an end sigmoid colostomy, who are dextrous, mentally alert, and who have enjoyed regular bowel habits prior to their illness. Training by approved personnel should commence six weeks post-operatively and after the perineal wound has healed. Irrigation is performed daily at a regular time for four weeks and thereafter every second day. The equipment consists of:

1. a water bag, connecting tube with regulating flow clamp and an attached cone (Figure 4.6);
2. a long plastic pouch opened at both ends.

The water bag is filled with 1000–1500 mL of warm tap water which is elevated to shoulder height so as to enable the water to run through the tubing in order to eliminate any airlock. The patient may sit or stand. The pouch is applied over the stoma, with its long end placed in the toilet (Colour Plate 4).

The lubricated cone is introduced through the open end of the pouch and is gently inserted in the direction of the

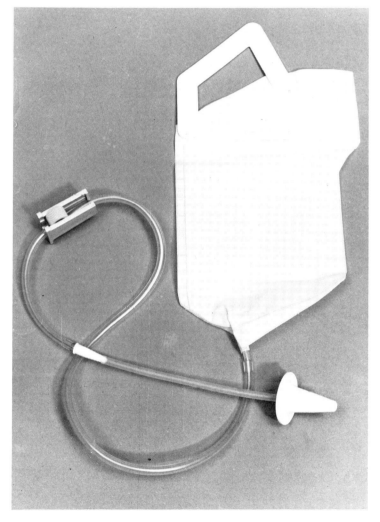

Fig. 4.6 Colostomy irrigation set

colostomy lumen (Colour Plate 5). The water should run for five to seven minutes, and then the cone is removed and the faeces emptied into the toilet. A minimal capacity pouch is applied after a variable interval when the patient feels evacuation is complete.

Potential problems
1.   Difficulties with water inflow may be due to:
     (a) An airlock caused by insufficient elevation of the water bag, or incorrect positioning of the cone.
     (b) Colostomy stenosis or paracolostomy hernia.
2.   Difficulties with faecal return may be due to colonic obstruction or a paracolostomy hernia.
3.   Evacuation between irrigations may be due to:
     (a) insufficient volume of water, that is less than 1500 mL;
     (b) dietary indescretions of which an increased alcohol intake is the commonest.

DIET

The patient may follow his usual dietary habits, although foods that are known to cause flatulence should be avoided. Constipation may be a problem, in which case simple measures such as increasing fluid intake and a high fibre diet may be helpful. Persistent constipation or diarrhoea may have an organic cause for which a medical opinion should be sought.

COLOSTOMY COMPLICATIONS

Skin excoriation (Colour Plate 6)
This common complication is due to faeces being in prolonged contact with the peristomal skin, which in turn may be due to:

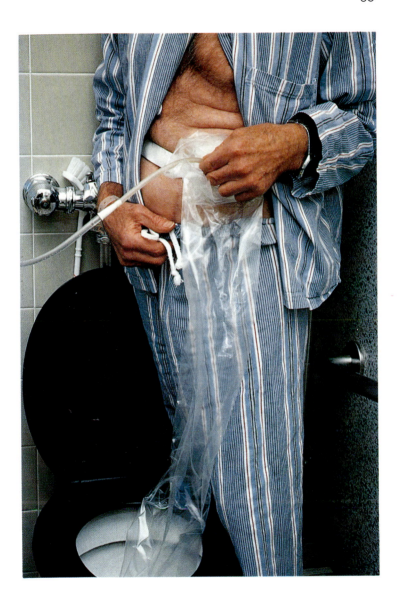

Colour Plate 4   Long bag applied

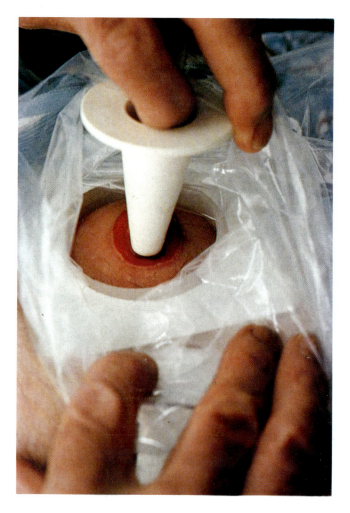

Colour Plate 5 Lubricated cone inserted

CHAPTER 5

Management of an Ileostomy

The change to a permanent appliance is made during convalescence, and several appliances may have to be tried before final selection.

Ileal fluid is irritating to skin, consequently the use of a skin barrier (such as Stomahesive or karaya gum) is recommended. Some appliances incorporate such a barrier.

Ileostomy pouches are usually changed every three to seven days. Because of the fluid nature of the faeces, it is desirable for them to be drainable.

ILEOSTOMY APPLIANCES

Before the development of plastics, ileostomy appliances consisted of an array of home-made boxes, absorbent pads and dressings. The inadequate fit of these over the ileostomy invariably resulted in leakage of ileal fluid onto the abdominal wall with consequent troublesome excoriation.

In 1944 Keonig devised a rubber appliance which revolutionised stomal care. The pouch was held onto the skin with a latex preparation. The development of the Keonig pouch coincided with that of plastics, and though rubber still remains popular, disposable lightweight appliances have taken over.

TYPES OF APPLIANCES

Disposable

These appliances are available in different sizes, shapes and colours to suit individual build and preference. They may be emptied during the day, and the complete unit disposed of every three to seven days. Basically there are four possible variations in design.

1. Colour and texture — a variety of patterned and opaque pouches are available (Figure 5.1).
2. Length of pouch — a person with a short torso may prefer a small pouch (Figure 5.2).
3. Pre-cut aperture — these are particularly useful to patients with poor eyesight or those with physical or mental impairment (Figure 5.3).
4. Skin barrier — some appliances already incorporate a skin barrier (Figure 5.4).

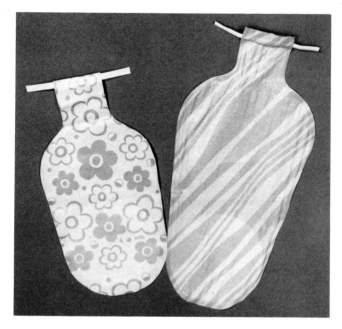

Fig. 5.1 Ileostomy appliances: different patterns

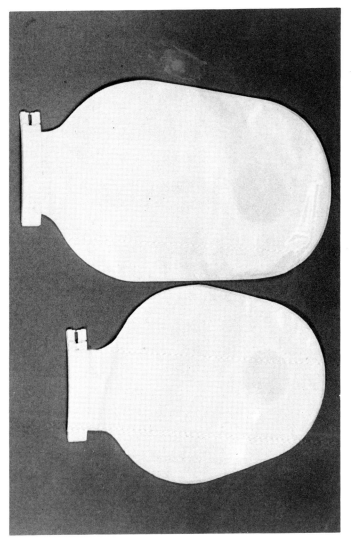

Fig. 5.2   Ileostomy appliances: different lengths

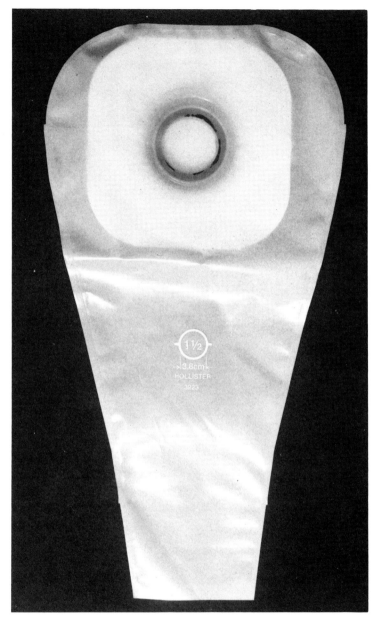

Fig. 5.3   Ileostomy pouch: pre-cut aperture

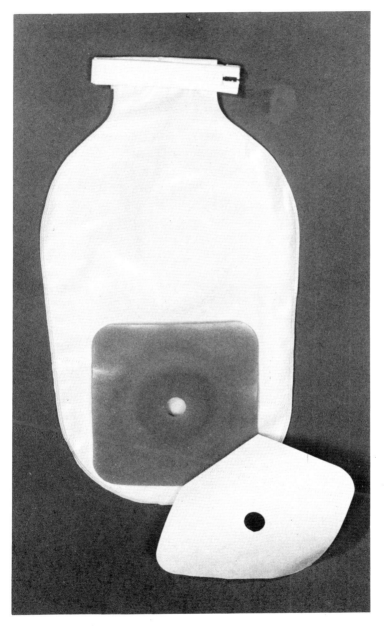

Fig. 5.4   Ileostomy appliance incorporating skin barrier

Non-disposable

These consist of a rubber pouch and flange. The flange is fitted to the skin using either a skin bond cement or double-sided adhesive plaster. Sometimes a skin barrier product is used as well (Figure 5.5). The flange is usually removed, cleaned and replaced once a week. The rubber pouch fits onto the flange and is provided with a drainage outlet. The pouch is changed every two to three days, and is used again after careful washing. Alternatively, a plastic or vinyl pouch may be fitted to the flange.

The flange is available in different sizes to ensure a secure fit. Pressure ulceration of the stoma may occur in which case a small karaya washer may be used between the ileostomy and the flange to prevent such ulceration.

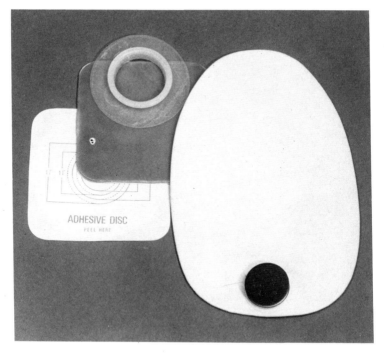

Fig. 5.5   Non-disposable ileostomy appliance

SKIN BARRIERS

Peristomal skin must be protected from ileal discharge. Adequate protection is the best prophylaxis against skin excoriation. There are various products available to protect the skin immediately adjacent to the ileostomy, and the peristomal skin in general.

Peristomal skin barriers

Basically there are two different types:
1. those providing a thin protective film, such as sprays, gels, wipe on swabs and paint (Figure 5.6); and
2. those providing a thick protective barrier. Most of these are ready-made wafers (Figure 5.7) such as Stomahesive, Reliaseal, Collyseals, Curaguard, and karaya. In hot weather, these wafers may soften, lose their efficiency and require changing more frequently.

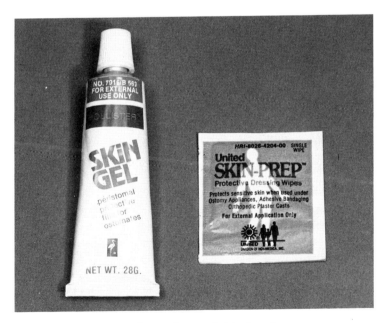

Fig. 5.6 Peristomal skin barriers

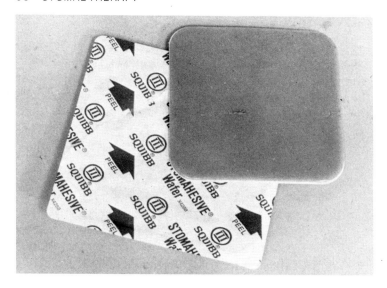

Fig. 5. 7   Ileostomy skin barrier (Stomahesive ®)

Barriers for the immediate peristomal skin
Some ileostomates prefer to use a small protective washer to provide a seal immediately around the stoma.

ILEOSTOMY COMPLICATIONS

There are many ileostomy complications, however, only those relevant to stomal care will be discussed.

Skin excoriation
This is the commonest complication. It is due to ileal fluid coming into contact with the skin which in turn may be due to a number of factors.
1. An inappropriate appliance or the incorrect use of an appliance are the commonest causes of excoriation. Sometimes the problem is very simple and easily remedied. For example, the aperture may have been cut too large, allowing leakage over the immediate peristomal skin.

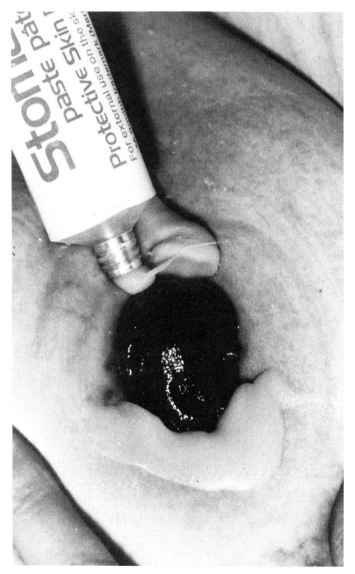

Fig. 5.9   Filling paste in skin crease

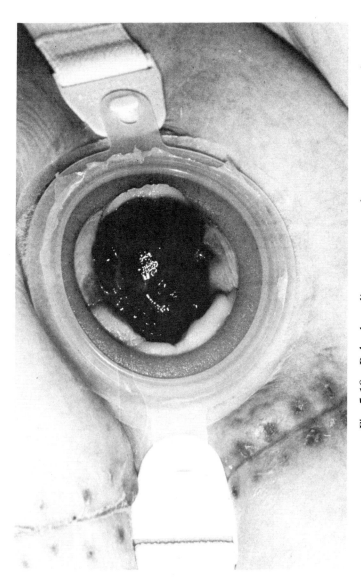

Fig. 5.10   Belted appliance to protrude stoma

Allergy of peristomal skin

The patient may be sensitive to the tape securing the appliance, the adhesive backing of the pouch or the type of skin barrier used. In such cases, use of the responsible product should be discontinued.

Pseudo-epitheliomatous hyperplasia (Figure 5.11)

In this condition, the mucosa appears to encroach over the peristomal skin. This is due to chronic trauma or irritation. It may be treated either conservatively or by surgical excision. Conservative management includes the use of a protective paste over the affected area to allow it to heal.

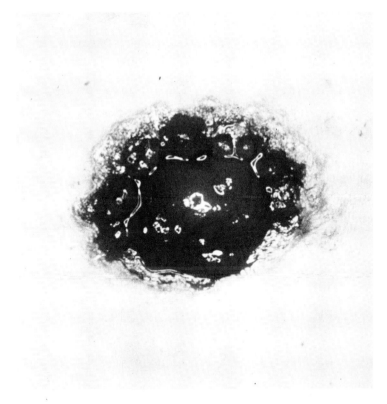

Fig. 5.11 Pseudo-epitheliomatous hyperplasia

Stomal ulcers

These are either due to pressure on the stoma from an ill-fitting appliance or recurrence of Crohn's disease. Pressure ulcers are easily diagnosed and are managed by the correct use of a suitable appliance. It is useful to apply Orohesive powder to the ulcer. This provides local pain relief and resolution of bleeding.

Obstruction

Small bowel obstruction occurs in up to thirty per cent of ileostomates. The obstruction is commonly due either to adhesions or to a food bolus. The patient usually complains of colicky abdominal pains and distension. The ileostomy output diminishes or stops and vomiting may occur. If the obstruction is partial, then the ileostomy output may in fact increase and become watery and straw-coloured. Patients with an obstruction are likely to become dehydrated and salt-depleted unless they are promptly treated by intravenous fluid and electrolyte replacement. Most respond to conservative treatment, however, surgery may be necessary in some to relieve the obstruction.

Dehydration

Occasionally patients may become dehydrated. This is likely to occur if the ileostomy output is high and especially in hot weather. An excessive loss of fluid and salt may lead to hypotension and muscle cramps. Mild episodes may be treated by increasing fluid and salt intake, however more severe episodes may require admission to hospital for intravenous fluid and electrolyte replenishment.

CHAPTER 6

The Continent Ileostomy

The continent ileostomy is an ileostomy which does not leak gas or faeces and over which an appliance need not be worn.

It was developed in 1969 by Professor N. G. Kock of Sweden. It is only used in a selected number of patients who have ulcerative colitis or familial polyposis coli. It is not used in patients with Crohn's disease.

Basically it consists of a terminal ileal reservoir and a valve which prevents the escape of gas and faeces. The reservoir is constructed by the anastomosis of two or three loops of small intestine (Figure 6.1).

The valve (nipple valve) is constructed by proximal invagination of the terminal ileum. Basically it functions as a one-way valve: as the pressure rises, the lips of the valve are brought together thus preventing the escape of gas and faeces (Figure 6.2).

During the operation, the surgeon leaves a wide-bore catheter indwelling into the reservoir (Figure 6.3). This catheter is left in for a period of three or four weeks post-operatively. Its purpose is to drain gas and faeces so as not to put any tension on the anastomotic sutures of the reservoir. If there is such tension, the sutures might loosen and an intraperitoneal leakage of faeces might occur resulting in peritonitis.

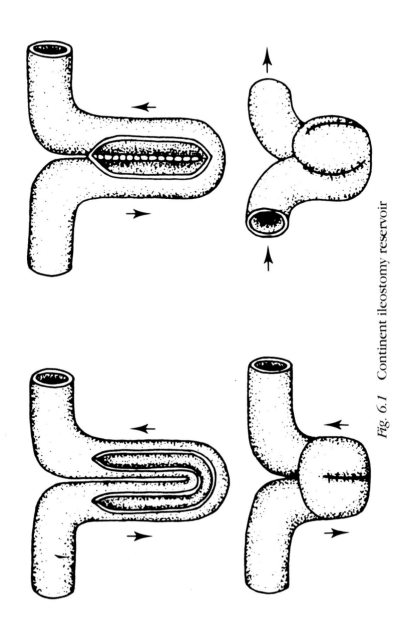

Fig. 6.1   Continent ileostomy reservoir

To ensure that the catheter does not slip out of the reservoir, it is common for it to be sutured to the peristomal skin and taped securely. If it accidentally falls out, the surgeon should be informed immediately so that he can promptly replace it in the reservoir.

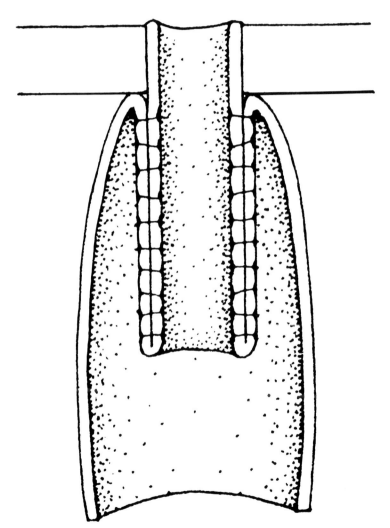

Fig. 6.2   Continent ileostomy valve

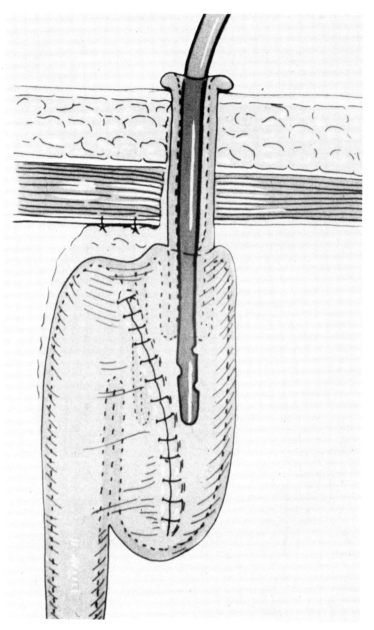

Fig. 6.3   Catheter left indwelling

POST-OPERATIVE CARE OF THE CATHETER

Position of the catheter
It is important to ensure that the catheter is not kinked (Figure 6.4). This may be done by placing a rolled gauze under the catheter. It is usual for the catheter to be connected to a bag or bottle.

Free-drainage
From the first post-operative day, the catheter should be very gently irrigated with normal saline solution at regular intervals to ensure that its tip is not blocked with a blood clot or with faeces. Should there be any concern regarding the patency of the catheter, then the surgeon should be notified in case the catheter needs changing.

Changing the catheter
Three to four weeks post-operatively, the surgeon usually changes the catheter and instructs the patient on self-catheterisation.

Self-catheterisation
Initially the patient may be instructed to empty the reservoir every three to four hours, however, over the next three to four months the interval is gradually increased until the reservoir is emptied three to four times daily. The patient is instructed to use a wide-bore well lubricated catheter (Figure 6.5). He or she should gently introduce the catheter into the ileostomy, past the valve, until gas or faeces pass into the tube (Figure 6.6). The catheter is then gently pushed in and out until the reservoir is empty. It is usual for the patient to irrigate the reservoir with 30 to 50 mL of water to ensure that it is completely empty. Following this the catheter is removed and the patient applies a small dressing over the ileostomy to absorb any mucous secreted.

Diet
The patient may eat a normal diet, however stringy vegetables, fruit piths and nuts should be avoided to prevent food blockage.

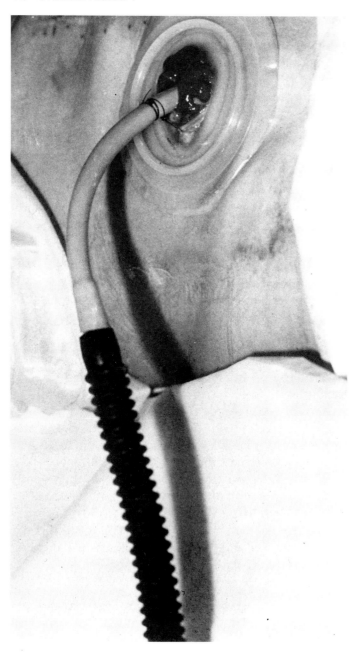

Fig. 6.4   Ensure that the catheter is not kinked

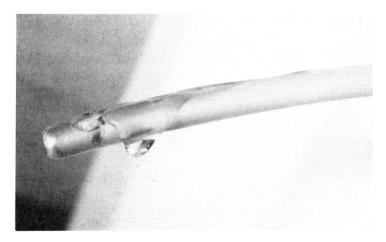

Fig. 6.5   Wide-bore lubricated catheter

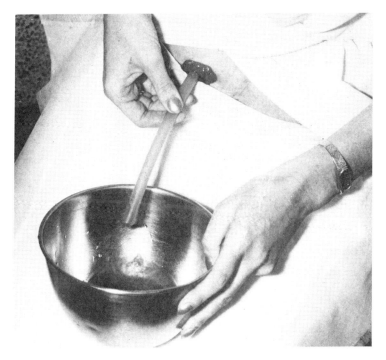

Fig. 6.6   Placing the catheter into the ileostomy

COMPLICATIONS

There are several complications of the continent ileostomy, however only those pertinent to nursing care will be considered.

Slipping of the valve

In some patients, the valve slips out (or dessuscepts) (Figure 6.7), in which case the patient will leak gas and faeces. Furthermore, he or she may have difficulty in passing the catheter into the reservoir. If this should happen, it is important not to use force to try and pass the catheter. The surgeon should be advised immediately and appropriate steps will then be taken. These usually involve re-operation to re-construct the valve.

Diarrhoea

Occasionally patients complain of severe diarrhoea with or without abdominal pain. This is often due to an inflammation of the reservoir which has been attributed to bacterial overgrowth. Medical attention should be sought.

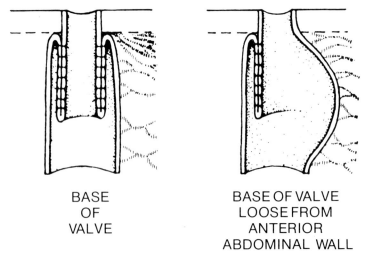

BASE
OF
VALVE

BASE OF VALVE
LOOSE FROM
ANTERIOR
ABDOMINAL WALL

Fig. 6.7 Dessuscepted (slipped) valve

CHAPTER 7

Temporary Stomata

TEMPORARY COLOSTOMY

A temporary colostomy may be necessary to divert faeces away from the left colon. The principle indications for this have been discussed in Chapter 1.

Many transverse colostomies are supported by a rod in the immediate post-operative period (Figure 7.1). There are many different types of rods, some of which are illustrated in Figure 7.2. The aim is to fit the rod into the pouch without trauma to the bowel (Figure 7.3). An appliance with a flexible backing is useful to enable manoeuvrability. If the rod has been sutured in place, then the aperture of the appliance must be cut to incorporate the rod. The decision to remove the rod is made by the surgeon, and it is customary for this to be done within seven to ten days of the operation (Figure 7.4)

LONG-TERM MANAGEMENT OF A TEMPORARY TRANSVERSE COLOSTOMY

The type of appliance used depends on the volume and nature of the output. This in turn will depend on the segment of transversed colon exteriorised. Thus, the output will be higher and more fluid the more proximal the segment. If the colostomy has a high output, then a drainable appliance is preferred (as with an ileostomy). However, if the output is low and thick in consistency, the patient may prefer a closed end appliance (as with a permanent end sigmoid colostomy). When there is a high output, a protective skin barrier is often used.

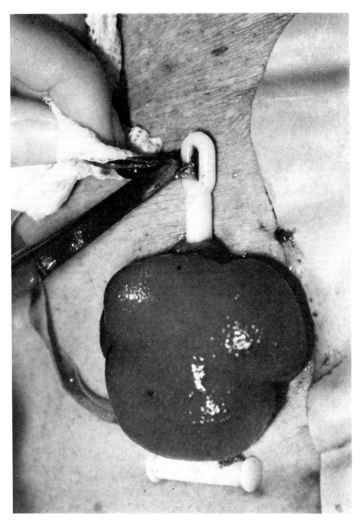

Fig. 7.1   Transverse colostomy supported by a rod

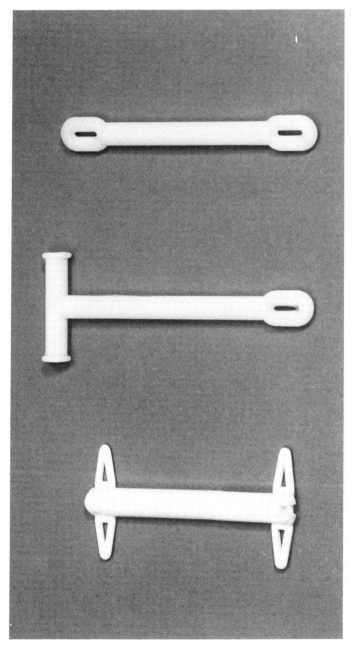

Fig. 7.2   Different types of rods

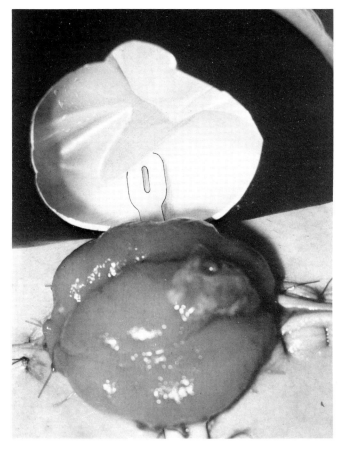

Fig. 7.3 Fitting the rod into the pouch

COMPLICATIONS OF A TRANSVERSE COLOSTOMY

Skin excoriation

The principles of management have been outlined in Chapters 4 and 5.

Prolapse

This complication occurs relatively frequently (Colour Plate 9) and is difficult to manage. With gentle pressure it is usually easy to reduce the prolapse, however, it invariably recurs. The only satisfactory method of dealing with this problem is to close the colostomy. Until this occurs, however, it may be difficult to apply the pouch over the prolapsed stoma. Certain measures may be taken to facilitate application.

1. The use of a cold pack to the prolapsed segment may help its reduction.
2. The prolapse may reduce spontaneously when the patient lies back.
3. Enlarging the aperture of the appliance.

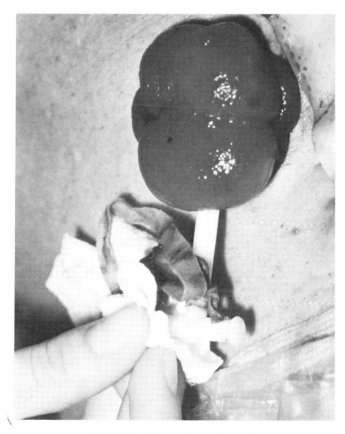

Fig. 7.4   Removing the rod

MANAGEMENT OF A LOOP ILEOSTOMY

A loop ileostomy is constructed by exteriorising a loop of terminal ileum at a site selected as for an end ileostomy. The ileum is then opened transversely and this results in a pro-truding functioning end and a flat defunctioned end (Figure 7.5).

A loop ileostomy, like a loop transverse colostomy is usually used when the distal colon needs to be rested (or defunctioned).

The management of a loop ileostomy is the same as an end ileostomy, however, in the immediate post-operative period the appliance has to be fitted over a rod as with a loop transverse colostomy (Colour Plate 10).

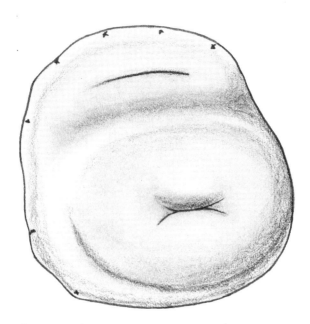

Fig. 7.5 Loop ileostomy: note protruding functional end

MANAGEMENT OF A CAECOSTOMY

As indicated in Chapter 1, a caecostomy is usually performed to defunction a distal colonic obstruction or anastomosis. The procedure has not been widely employed because it is difficult to care for a caecostomy post-operatively.

There are two ways of constructing a caecostomy:

1. *Tube caecostomy* (Figure 7.6)
    In this technique a large bore catheter is introduced into the caecum and exteriorised through a stab wound.

2. *Immediate mucocutaneous suturing* (Colour Plate 11)
    In this technique an incision is made into the caecum which is sutured directly to the skin.

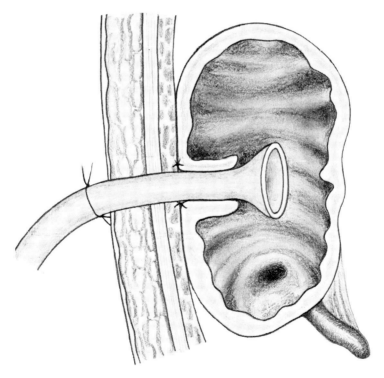

Fig. 7.6 Tube caecostomy

CARE OF A TUBE CAECOSTOMY

The principle aim is to keep the tube patent by regular, gentle irrigation with tap-water. As a rule, the surgeon will remove the tube once the distal obstruction has been relieved. This usually results in a faecal fistula over which a pouch together with a protective barrier (similar to that used for an ileostomy) should be worn. Provided there is no distal obstruction the fistula usually closes spontaneously.

CARE OF A MUCOCUTANEOUS CAECOSTOMY

It is important to site a caecostomy as carefully as any other stoma. The effluent from a caecostomy is very liquid, odorous and excoriating to skin. it is therefore important to take appropriate measures to protect the peristomal skin. These include careful siting, protective barriers and drainable pouches. Basically the same principles apply to the care of a caecostomy as apply to an ileostomy.

CHAPTER 8

Urinary Diversion Stomas

There are many ways of diverting urine from the bladder. These include ileal conduits, colonic conduits and exteriorising the ureters themselves to the abdominal wall (ureterostomy).

In some patients urine is diverted by anastomosing the ureters to the sigmoid colon (ureterosigmoidostomy). In these patients there is no need for a stoma, as an intact rectum provides continence for both urine and faeces (Figure 8.1).

The principle indications for urinary diversion are carcinoma of the bladder and certain neurogenic disorders of the bladder. The most common method of diversion is via an ileal conduit.

ILEAL CONDUIT STOMA

The bladder may or may not have been resected (cystectomy). A segment of terminal ileum is isolated with its own vascular supply and small intestinal continuity is restored (Figure 8.2). The proximal end of this isolated segment is oversewn and the ureters anastomosed to the conduit — usually in an end-to-side fashion. The other end of the conduit is exteriorised as a conventional ileostomy (Figure 8.3). The conduit is not a reservoir and urine should flow without obstruction into an appliance.

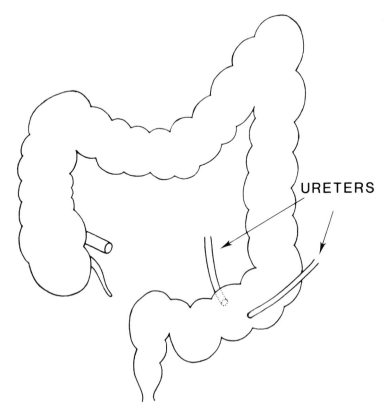

Fig. 8.1   Uretero-sigmoid urinary diversion

SITING

The site is chosen pre-operatively using the same principles as those for an end ileostomy.

MANAGEMENT

It is common for the surgeon to pass fine catheters into the ureters to allow the anastomosis between the ureters and

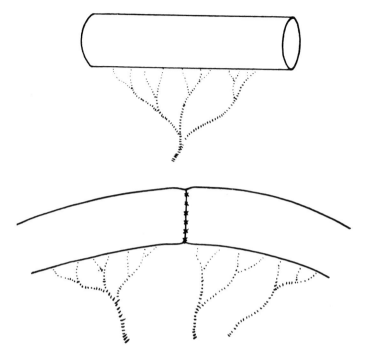

Fig. 8.2 Loop ileum isolated, intestinal continuity restored

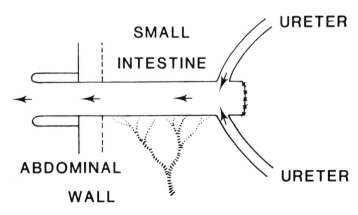

Fig. 8.3 Ileal conduit: ureters anastomosed to proximal end, distal end exteriorised

the small intestine to heal adequately (Figure 8.4). These catheters fall out of their own accord ten to fourteen days post-operatively, and should not be disturbed. It is common for mucous to be secreted by the mucosa of the small intestinal conduit.

APPLIANCES

Several are available, some incorporating a skin barrier, the use of which is recommended. Pouches are changed every three to five days and have a tap device to facilitate drainage of the urine (Figure 8.5).

Some patients prefer to have continuous drainage at night in which case suitable connections are available (Figure 8.6). Continuous drainage is also used in the post-operative period.

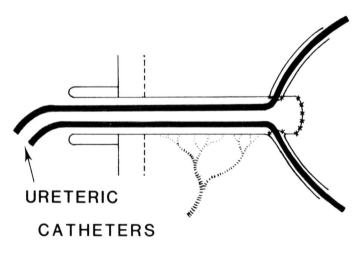

URETERIC

CATHETERS

Fig. 8.4(a)   Ureteric catheters

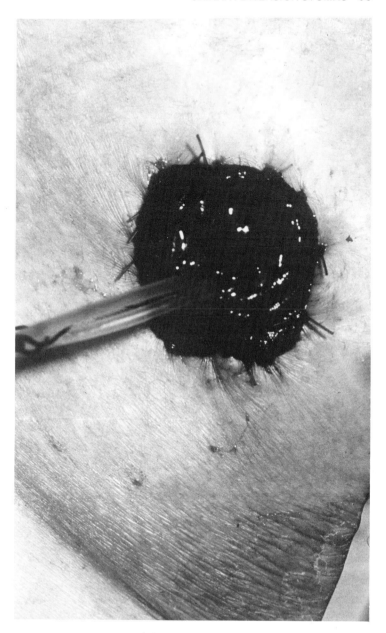

Fig. 8.4(b) Ureteric catheter

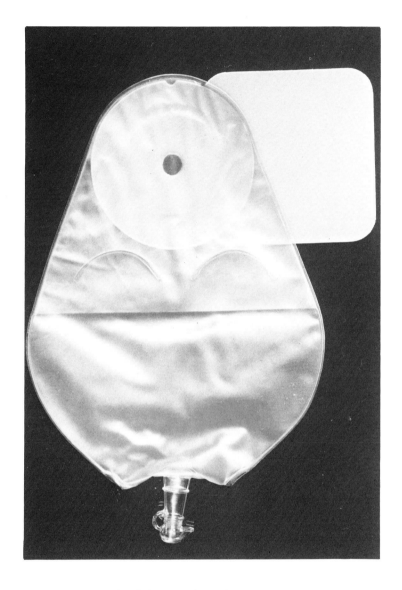

Fig. 8.5 Pouch with tap device

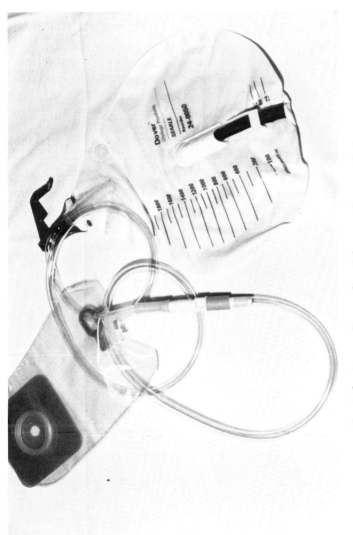

Fig. 8.6   An appliance fitted for continuous drainage

TYPES OF APPLIANCES

Disposable appliances

Different shapes and sizes are available and most incorporate a non-return anti-reflux valve. There are three main variations in design.

1. Size of pouch — large volume pouches are available.
2. Pre-cut apertures — these may be useful for patients with poor eyesight or who lack manual dexterity.
3. Skin barriers — some appliances already incorporate a skin barrier.

Non-disposable appliances

These are very similar to ileostomy non-disposable appliances except that they have a tap outlet. When using a non-disposable appliance a skin barrier should also be used (Figure 8.7).

COMPLICATIONS

General complications

Complications that may occur with a stoma may also occur with a urinary diversion stoma. These include necrosis, stenosis, haematoma, retraction and poor siting. These have all been dealt with in Chapter 3.

Specific complications

There are however certain complications specific to a urinary diversion stoma. Only those relevant to stoma care will be discussed.

1. *Urinary tract infections* These occur relatively frequently. If the patient complains of cloudy and odourous urine, a urine sample for culture and sensitivity should be taken. This is done by passing a sterile catheter into the conduit. During this procedure caution should be taken not to perforate the conduit by forcible introduction. A strict sterile protocol should be observed. Once the catheter is in the conduit the first

10 mL of urine should be discarded to avoid contamination of the specimen. In some centres a double lumen catheter is used to avoid contamination. Basically this consists of two catheters one within the other.

It is advisable to investigate the patient by intravenous pyelography (IVP) and contrast X-rays of the conduit (conduitogram) to assess emptying and ureteric reflux. After assessment the patient should be treated with an appropriate antibiotic, and should increase his or her fluid intake. In addition the patient should wear disposable appliances which are emptied frequently to prevent urinary stasis. A pouch incorporating an anti-reflux device should be used.

2. *Peristomal urinary stagnation* If urine stagnates around the stoma, then constant pooling of urine may result in:

(a) uric acid crystals being deposited over the stoma and peristomal skin;
(b) peristomal skin scarring (Figure 8.8);
(c) stomal stenosis (Figure 8.8).

The first two conditions may be treated conservatively, but the third condition, stomal stenosis, may require surgical revision.

Conservative management of uric acid crystals consists of the application of a one to-one solution of vinegar (acetic acid) and water to the affected areas several times a day. It is equally important to prevent pooling of urine. Disposable appliances should be used and changed daily. It may also be helpful to have the appliance on continuous drainage during the night. The urine should be acidified by the patient taking oral ascorbic acid. Occasionally, the patient may need to be admitted to hospital.

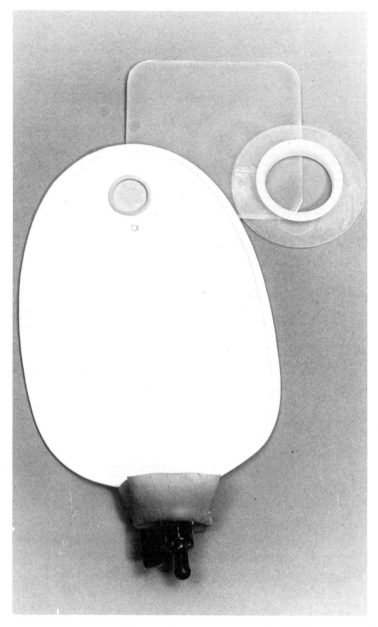

Fig. 8.7   Non-disposable appliance with skin barrier

CHAPTER 9

Quality of Life

Today ostomates go unnoticed in our community. There are no external features which distinguish an ostomate from the rest of us. Gone are the days when a person with a stoma had to lead a closeted and restricted life. There is no reason why an ostomate cannot realise the same ambitions that other people aspire to. Numerous surveys have shown that most ostomates lead full and active working, sporting, social and sexual lives. They live and work in every stratum of our society and some have distinguished themselves in sport, entertainment, politics and in the professions. Some have even attained the heights of Olympian sportsmen and women.

These achievements, however, have not been attained by accident. Over the past three decades major advances have been made in surgical techniques and appliances which have simplified the day-to-day care of a stoma. However, the most significant contributions have been made by stomal therapy nurses and self-help groups and associations. These two groups of people have offered prospective ostomates detailed and reliable information, thus removing the main source of anxiety, namely fear of the unknown. The support given is extended well into the post-operative period when patients return to their home environment to resume their normal lives.

Several questions are frequently asked by the prospective ostomate and in this chapter an attempt is made to answer the most common ones.

DIET

As a rule, there should be no dietary restrictions whatsoever, however, foods which are known to disagree with the ostomate should be avoided. Most ileostomates should be encouraged to chew their food adequately and to eat fibrous (or stringy) items in moderation, furthermore, they should avoid corn kernals and nuts which may cause a food bolus obstruction. In hot weather ileostomates should increase their fluid and salt intake to prevent dehydration and salt losses. An excessive alcohol intake may cause diarrhoea and should be avoided.

FLATUS AND ODOUR

Many ostomates are anxious to know whether flatus and odour will be an embarrassment to them. Simple reassurance that modern disposable appliances are odour proof should allay their fears. Further protection against odour may be obtained by using deodorants which are available for that purpose. Some deodorants may be chemically irritant to the stoma and should be used with caution. Foods known to cause flatulence should be avoided, if however, excessive flatulence should continue, then charcoal tablets may be taken orally. Alternatively, natural yoghurt has been recommended by some.

CLOTHES

Clothes, fashion and external appearances are a frequent source of anxiety to many prospective ostomates who fear that their appliances will bulge and become noticeable in public. Consequently most ostomates think that they have to wear loose fitting garments which will mask their appliances. This view, however, is not correct. With the wide variety of appliances now available, ostomates can choose to wear any style of clothing including tight-fitting and waisted garments. The same applies to corsets, underwear and swimwear. Most ostomates today keep up with the latest fashion and there is no way of externally distinguishing them from the rest of the community. This has to be emphasised pre-operatively to allay anxieties.

SPORT

Like any other person, an ostomate should be encouraged to participate in any sport of his or her choice. Body contact sports are sometimes avoided, but the decision to do so should be made by the individual since there is no reason why an ostomate should not participate in such sports. Similarly, there is no reason to avoid swimming and water sports. Simple measures such as emptying the pouch beforehand and securing it with waterproof tape are all that are necessary. A smaller pouch is sometimes preferred for water sports.

TRAVELLING

A stoma should not prevent a person from travelling by air, sea or any other form of transport. If an extended trip is taken, adequate supplies should either be carried or information sought on supplies available at the various places intended to be visited. It is wise to carry some supplies in hand luggage in case other luggage is lost. When driving a car, some ostomates are concerned that wearing a seat belt may injure their stoma. If the seat belt abutts onto the stoma then they should wear a small protective pad. If this small precaution is taken then the ostomate should find no difficulties with wearing a seat belt.

SHOWERING AND BATHING

The decision whether or not to shower or bathe with the appliance on should be made by the individual. If the ostomate wishes to keep the appliance on during showering, waterproof tape may be used.

INFECTION

Some ostomates are concerned that skin infection may occur should faeces come into contact with the abdominal wall. These fears should be discounted.

LEAKAGE

A common question and source of anxiety to most ostomates is the possibility of the appliance leaking in public. Although leakage may occur, it should happen rarely if the appliance has been properly managed and regularly emptied. Nevertheless, it is advisable to carry spare equipment at all times. The first sign of leakage is often odour indicating an escape of gas. This should alert the ostomate to check the security of the pouch.

TELLING FRIENDS AND RELATIVES

There are no obvious features that distinguish an ostomate from any other member of the community. This should be impressed on all ostomates so that their decision to tell friends and relatives of their condition should be based on personal preferance.

SEXUALITY

Another area that causes concern to patients is their ability to perform sexually after their surgery. Patients are often unable to imagine what they will look like after surgery and furthermore some imagine that their genitalia will be disfigured. In the past the subject was usually neglected, however, with the emancipation in recent years of society's views on sexuality, greater emphasis is now being placed on this important subject.

Quite naturally patients are often embarrassed to discuss their sexual lives, and it is up to the surgeon and stomal therapy nurse to establish a good rapport with the patient in order to open up discussion. One important point to remember is that many people in the community have little concept of their sexual anatomy, therefore, it may be worthwhile to demonstrate with a model or drawing exactly what the surgery entails and how it will *not* affect the genitalia. It may also be worthwhile to include in these discussions the patient's partner who is often as equally confused and anxious.

A stoma should not interfere with sexual enjoyment, however, some patients develop sexual problems which may either be organic or psychological.

Organic

In males, the most common problem is impotence. This is often related to the type of surgery which has been performed. In patients with a rectal carcinoma, wide excision of the rectum often results in damage to pelvic nerves which subserve sexual function. The incidence of impotence in these patients is higher than in patients with ulcerative colitis in whom a more limited dissection is sufficient. In some males even though erection is achieved ejaculation does not occur.

In females undergoing pelvic dissection the most common complaint is dyspareunia (pain during intercourse) which has been attributed to pelvic adhesions.

Patients with an organic cause for their sexual problems should not be neglected. Many can be helped to enjoy other ways of achieving sexual satisfaction. The use and availability of sexual aids should be discussed openly, and sometimes consultation with a sexual therapist may be heplful.

Psychological

A major fear held by most patients is that they will be less attractive and desirable after the operation. This fear is accentuated by their self-image: they regard themselves as scarred for life, as being only half a man or woman and so on. In addition some patients are anxious that somehow people will know that they have a stoma and that this will restrict their ability to meet suitable partners. They also naturally wonder whether their appliance will leak during sexual intercourse and whether the stoma will be repugnant to their partner.

These fears are very real and should not be dismissed. Time, patience and effort in counselling both partners is essential. It is important to stress to the patient that the majority of ostomates enjoy sexual intercourse as much, and as often, as the rest of the community. Some patients, especially, ileostomates who had suffered chronic illness before their operation, found in fact that their general well being after surgery increased their sexual satisfaction.

A major concern to some patients is the possibility that the appliance may leak during sexual intercourse. This occurs very infrequently and a simple but often unnecessary precaution is to empty the pouch beforehand. Some ostomates may be concerned that a clear plastic appliance may deter their partners, in which case a decorated pouch or a pouch-cover may be worn. Variations in sexual positions should not be discouraged and the patient should be reassured that the stoma cannot be injured during sexual intercourse.

PREGNANCY

Many patients fear that they will not be able to have children after their operation. This is in fact not correct. Ostomates can become pregnant and deliver normal babies per vaginum. Many are concerned that pregnancy may somehow injure the stoma or interfere with its function. They should be gently reassured that this is not the case.

In conclusion the prospective ostomate is often faced with many questions and anxieties. Many of these are based on fear of the unknown and misinformation. With a coordinated team approach, most of these fears can be overcome to allow the patient to lead and enjoy a fulfilling life.